The Blooming Womb Cookbook:

Delicious & Nourishing Recipes for Optimizing Women's Fertility

Jennifer Willeford

Table of contents

Introduction

In the pursuit of starting or expanding a family, fertility becomes a vital aspect of a woman's life. The desire to conceive and bear a child is deeply ingrained in human nature, and for some women, achieving optimal fertility may require certain dietary adjustments. This is where the concept of a fertility diet comes into play. A fertility diet refers to a strategic and intentional approach to nutrition that aims to enhance reproductive health and increase the chances of conception for women.

Throughout history, various cultures have recognized the connection between diet and fertility. Today, with advancements in scientific research, we have a deeper understanding of how specific nutrients can influence reproductive function. A fertility diet incorporates a range of foods that provide essential vitamins, minerals, antioxidants, and other beneficial compounds that promote hormonal balance, support egg quality, regulate menstrual cycles, and create a favorable environment for conception.

It is important to note that a fertility diet is not a guarantee of pregnancy, nor does it replace medical interventions for infertility. However, it can be a complementary approach that supports overall reproductive health and maximizes the chances of conceiving naturally or in conjunction with assisted reproductive technologies.

The fundamental principles of a fertility diet revolve around consuming whole, nutrient-dense foods while minimizing or eliminating potentially harmful substances. This diet emphasizes a balanced intake of macronutrients (carbohydrates, proteins, and fats) and micronutrients (vitamins and minerals) to optimize reproductive function. Additionally, it encourages the consumption of foods that are low in added sugars, refined carbohydrates, and unhealthy fats, as these may negatively impact fertility.

One of the key factors in a fertility diet is maintaining a healthy weight. Both being underweight and overweight can have adverse effects on fertility. Excessive body fat can disrupt hormone production and ovulation, while insufficient body fat can lead to hormonal imbalances and irregular menstrual cycles. Therefore, a fertility diet focuses on achieving and maintaining a healthy body weight through a well-rounded and wholesome eating plan.

Another crucial aspect of a fertility diet is the inclusion of specific nutrients that are known to play a role in reproductive health. For example, antioxidants such as vitamins C and E, beta-carotene, and selenium help protect the reproductive organs from oxidative damage and promote sperm and egg quality. Omega-3 fatty acids, found in fatty fish, flaxseeds, and walnuts, are beneficial for regulating hormones and reducing inflammation. Additionally, adequate intake of iron, folate, and vitamin B12 is vital for healthy ovulation and embryo development.

The fertility diet also takes into account the importance of hydration and encourages women to consume an adequate amount of water daily. Staying properly hydrated supports the production of cervical mucus, which plays a crucial role in creating a favorable environment for sperm to travel through the reproductive tract.

While the concept of a fertility diet may seem overwhelming at first, it is important to approach it with a balanced mindset. Rather than strict rules or rigid meal plans, it is best to view it as a framework for making informed food choices that support reproductive health. Experimenting with fertility-friendly recipes can be an enjoyable way to incorporate the necessary nutrients into your daily meals.

In this comprehensive guide, we will explore a variety of fertility diet recipes that are both nutritious and delicious. From breakfast options rich in fertility-boosting ingredients to nourishing lunch and dinner recipes, and even snacks and desserts that satisfy your cravings while supporting your reproductive goals, we have curated a collection of recipes to inspire and guide you on your fertility journey.

Remember, everyone's fertility journey is unique, and it's essential to consult with a healthcare professional or a registered dietitian to personalize your fertility diet based on your specific needs and health conditions. So, let's embark on this culinary exploration of fertility diet recipes and take a step closer to nurturing your reproductive health and achieving your dreams of motherhood.

Chapter 1

Understanding Fertility and Diet

Fertility, the ability to conceive and have a healthy pregnancy, is a topic of great importance for many individuals and couples. While fertility is influenced by various factors, such as age, underlying health conditions, and genetics, research has shown that diet and lifestyle choices can also significantly impact reproductive health. In this comprehensive chapter, we will explore the link between diet and fertility, discuss key nutrients that can boost fertility, and examine lifestyle factors that affect fertility.

1.1 The Link between Diet and Fertility

The connection between diet and fertility has gained significant attention in recent years, with numerous studies highlighting the potential impact of dietary choices on reproductive health. A healthy, balanced diet plays a crucial role in optimizing fertility potential for both men and women.

1.1.1 Weight and Fertility:

Weight management is an important aspect of fertility. Both being overweight and underweight can have negative effects on reproductive function. Obesity has been linked to hormonal imbalances, irregular menstrual cycles, and ovulation disorders in women. In men, obesity can lead to decreased sperm quality and quantity. On the other hand, being underweight can disrupt hormone production, leading to irregular or absent menstrual cycles in women and reduced sperm production in men. Therefore, achieving and maintaining a healthy weight through a balanced diet and regular exercise is crucial for improving fertility outcomes.

1.1.2 Insulin Resistance and Fertility:

Insulin resistance, a condition where the body's cells become less responsive to insulin, has been associated with fertility issues, particularly in women with polycystic ovary syndrome (PCOS). PCOS is a common hormonal disorder characterized by irregular menstrual cycles, high levels of androgens (male hormones), and small cysts on the ovaries. Insulin resistance can exacerbate the hormonal imbalances in PCOS, affecting ovulation and fertility. Consuming a diet that helps manage blood sugar levels and insulin resistance, such as a low glycemic index (GI) diet rich in whole grains, lean proteins, fruits, and vegetables, may benefit women with PCOS and enhance fertility.

1.2 Key Nutrients for Boosting Fertility

Certain nutrients have been found to play a crucial role in reproductive health and fertility. Including these key nutrients in your diet can help support optimal fertility outcomes.

1.2.1 Antioxidants

Antioxidants are compounds that help protect the body from oxidative stress, which can damage sperm and egg cells. Including a variety of antioxidant-rich foods in your diet can help promote fertility. Fruits such as berries (blueberries, strawberries, raspberries), citrus fruits (oranges, lemons), and pomegranates are excellent sources of antioxidants. Vegetables like spinach, kale, broccoli, and bell peppers also provide a range of antioxidants. Additionally, nuts such as walnuts and almonds, as well as legumes like beans and lentils, contain high levels of antioxidants and are beneficial for fertility.

1.2.2 Omega-3 Fatty Acids

Omega-3 fatty acids, specifically docosahexaenoic acid (DHA) and eicosapentaenoic acid (EPA), are essential for reproductive health. These fatty acids have been associated with improved hormone production, reduced inflammation, and enhanced blood flow to the reproductive organs. Including fatty fish like salmon, mackerel, and sardines in your diet can provide a good source of omega-3 fatty acids. Plant-based sources of omega-3s include chia seeds, flaxseeds, and walnuts.

1.2.3 Folate

Folate, also known as vitamin B9, is a crucial nutrient for both male and female fertility. It is essential for DNA synthesis,
cell division, and the healthy development of the neural tube in early pregnancy. Consuming foods rich in folate can support reproductive health. Leafy green vegetables like spinach and kale, lentils, avocado, and citrus fruits are excellent sources of folate.

1.2.4 Iron

Iron is an important mineral for reproductive health, particularly for women. Iron deficiency has been linked to ovulatory infertility and an increased risk of complications during pregnancy. Consuming iron-rich foods can help maintain adequate iron levels and support fertility. Lean meats, poultry, fish, spinach, beans, and fortified cereals are good sources of iron.

1.2.5 Zinc

Zinc is an essential mineral for male fertility as it plays a key role in sperm production and quality. Including zinc-rich foods in the diet can support reproductive health in men. Oysters, beef, lamb, pumpkin seeds, and chickpeas are excellent sources of zinc.

1.2.6 Vitamin D

Vitamin D deficiency has been associated with infertility and hormonal imbalances. Adequate vitamin D levels are important for both male and female fertility. The body can produce vitamin D through exposure to sunlight, but it can also be obtained from dietary sources. Fatty fish like salmon, fortified dairy products, and egg yolks are good sources of vitamin D.

1.3 Lifestyle Factors Affecting Fertility

In addition to diet, various lifestyle factors can impact fertility. Making positive lifestyle choices can enhance fertility outcomes and overall reproductive health.

1.3.1 Caffeine and Alcohol

High caffeine intake has been linked to delayed conception and an increased risk of miscarriage. It is advisable to limit caffeine consumption when trying to conceive. It is recommended to consume no more than 200-300 milligrams of caffeine per day, which is equivalent to about 1-2 cups of coffee. Similarly, excessive alcohol consumption can negatively affect fertility. It is best to limit alcohol intake or avoid it altogether when trying to conceive.

1.3.2 Smoking

Smoking has detrimental effects on fertility in both men and women. It can decrease sperm count, impair egg quality, and increase the risk of miscarriage and ectopic pregnancy. Quitting smoking is crucial for improving fertility outcomes.

1.3.3 Stress Management

Chronic stress can disrupt hormonal balance and interfere with reproductive function. High levels of stress can affect the hypothalamus, the part of the brain responsible for regulating hormone production. Engaging in stress-reducing activities such as regular exercise, meditation, yoga, and seeking support from loved ones or professionals can help manage stress levels and improve fertility.

1.3.4 Exercise

Regular physical activity is beneficial for overall health and fertility. Moderate exercise has been associated with improved fertility outcomes. However, excessive exercise or intense workouts can have a negative impact on fertility in some cases, particularly in women. It is important to maintain a balanced exercise routine and avoid excessive strain on the body.

Understanding the link between diet, key nutrients, and lifestyle factors is essential for optimizing fertility. While diet alone cannot guarantee fertility, adopting a healthy, balanced diet that includes key nutrients can positively impact reproductive health. Additionally, making positive lifestyle choices, such as managing weight, limiting caffeine and alcohol intake, quitting smoking, managing stress levels, and engaging in moderate exercise, can further support fertility outcomes. It is important to remember that fertility is a complex issue influenced by various factors, and individuals experiencing fertility challenges should seek guidance from healthcare professionals for a comprehensive evaluation and personalized recommendations. By prioritizing a healthy lifestyle and making informed dietary choices, individuals can increase their chances of achieving optimal reproductive health and enhancing fertility.

Chapter 2

Preparing for a Fertility Diet

When it comes to preparing for a pregnancy, one aspect that often gets overlooked is the importance of a healthy diet. A well-balanced and nutritious diet can significantly improve fertility and increase the chances of conception. This is where a fertility diet comes into play. A fertility diet focuses on consuming foods that promote reproductive health and support optimal hormone levels. In this article, we will discuss the key steps involved in preparing for a fertility diet, including consulting with a healthcare professional, assessing your current diet, and setting realistic goals.

2.1 Consulting with a Healthcare Professional

Before embarking on any dietary changes, it is crucial to consult with a healthcare professional, such as a fertility specialist or a registered dietitian who specializes in reproductive health. These professionals can provide personalized guidance based on your specific needs and medical history. They will help you understand the impact of diet on fertility and guide you through the process of preparing for a fertility diet.

During your consultation, the healthcare professional will evaluate your overall health and any underlying conditions that may affect your fertility. They may recommend specific tests to assess hormone levels, nutritional deficiencies, or any other factors that could hinder conception. By understanding your unique circumstances, they can offer tailored advice and create a personalized fertility diet plan.

2.2 Assessing Your Current Diet

To prepare for a fertility diet, it is essential to assess your current eating habits and identify areas that need improvement. Keeping a food diary for a week can be an effective way to track your daily intake. Note down everything you eat and drink, including portion sizes and cooking methods. This will provide valuable insights into your dietary patterns and help you identify potential areas for modification.

When assessing your current diet, pay attention to the following key factors:

2.2.1 Macronutrient Balance: A fertility diet should include a balanced combination of macronutrients - carbohydrates, proteins, and fats. Aim for a diet that provides adequate amounts of each macronutrient, as they all play a role in reproductive health. Ensure that your diet contains a variety of whole grains, lean proteins, and healthy fats.

2.2.2 Micronutrient Intake: Micronutrients, such as vitamins and minerals, are essential for reproductive function. Assess your intake of key fertility-promoting nutrients, including folate, zinc, iron, vitamin D, and omega-3 fatty acids. Consider incorporating more fertility-friendly foods that are rich in these nutrients, such as leafy greens, citrus fruits, nuts, seeds, and oily fish.

2.2.3 Hydration: Proper hydration is crucial for overall health, including fertility. Evaluate your daily fluid intake and make sure you are adequately hydrated. Water is the best choice, but you can also include herbal teas or infused water for variety. Minimize or eliminate sugary beverages and excessive caffeine, as they may negatively impact fertility.

2.2.4 Food Quality: Assess the quality of the foods you consume. Opt for whole, unprocessed foods whenever possible. Minimize your intake of processed and packaged foods, which often contain artificial additives, preservatives, and unhealthy trans fats. Choose organic produce and grass-fed or free-range animal products to reduce exposure to pesticides and hormones.

2.2.5 Lifestyle Habits: In addition to diet, lifestyle factors such as smoking, alcohol consumption, and physical activity can influence fertility. Assess these habits and consider making positive changes. Quit smoking, reduce alcohol intake, and engage in regular moderate exercise to optimize your reproductive health.

2.3 Setting Realistic Goals

Once you have assessed your current diet, it is important to set realistic goals that align with your fertility and health objectives. Setting attainable goals can help you stay motivated and make gradual changes to your eating habits. Consider the following steps when setting goals for your fertility diet:

2.3.1 Prioritize Nutrient-Rich Foods: Set a goal to incorporate more fertility-friendly foods into your diet. Focus on nutrient-rich options such as fruits, vegetables, whole grains, lean proteins, and healthy fats. Gradually replace processed and unhealthy foods with these nutritious alternatives.

2.3.2 Portion Control: Assess your portion sizes and aim for moderation. Overeating or undereating can both negatively impact fertility. Work with a healthcare professional or registered dietitian to determine appropriate portion sizes based on your individual needs.

2.3.3 Gradual Modifications: Instead of making drastic changes overnight, consider making gradual modifications to your diet. Set small, achievable goals that can be sustained over the long term. For example, start by incorporating one additional serving of vegetables into your daily meals and gradually increase the amount over time.

2.3.4 Meal Planning: Plan your meals in advance to ensure that you have a well-balanced and fertility-friendly diet. Set a goal to dedicate time each week to meal planning, grocery shopping, and preparing meals. This will help you stay organized and reduce the temptation to rely on unhealthy convenience foods.

2.3.5 Monitor Progress: Regularly monitor your progress to stay motivated and track your achievements. Keep a food diary or use smartphone apps to record your meals, track your nutrient intake, and monitor your portion sizes. This self-monitoring can provide valuable insights and help you identify areas for improvement.

Preparing for a fertility diet involves several key steps that can significantly improve your chances of conception. By consulting with a healthcare professional, assessing your current diet, and setting realistic goals, you can embark on a journey towards a healthier and more fertility-friendly lifestyle. Remember that the fertility diet is not a quick fix but a long-term commitment to nourishing your body for optimal reproductive health. Stay consistent, seek support when needed, and embrace the positive changes you make along the way.

Chapter 3

The Fertility Diet Guidelines

In recent years, there has been an increasing focus on the impact of nutrition on fertility. Many couples trying to conceive are now incorporating dietary changes into their lifestyle to enhance their chances of successful conception. The fertility diet is a comprehensive approach that emphasizes the consumption of whole foods, balancing macronutrients, ensuring adequate intake of micronutrients, and maintaining proper hydration. In this article, we will explore these guidelines in detail, providing valuable insights into how nutrition can play a crucial role in optimizing fertility.

3.1 Whole Foods vs. Processed Foods:

When it comes to fertility, the quality of the food we consume matters greatly. Whole foods, in their natural and unprocessed form, are rich in essential nutrients that promote reproductive health. On the other hand, processed foods, which are often high in added sugars, unhealthy fats, and artificial additives, can have a detrimental effect on fertility.

Whole foods include fruits, vegetables, whole grains, lean proteins, and healthy fats. These foods are packed with vitamins, minerals, antioxidants, and fiber that support hormonal balance and overall reproductive function. In contrast, processed foods such as sugary snacks, refined grains, and fast food can lead to insulin resistance, inflammation, and hormonal imbalances, which can negatively impact fertility.

Adopting a fertility diet involves replacing processed foods with whole foods whenever possible. Prioritizing fresh fruits and vegetables, whole grains like quinoa and brown rice, lean proteins like poultry and fish, and healthy fats from sources like avocados, nuts, and seeds can provide the body with the necessary nutrients to support reproductive health.

3.2 Balancing Macronutrients:

Macronutrients, including carbohydrates, proteins, and fats, are the building blocks of our diet and play a crucial role in fertility. Each macronutrient serves a specific purpose in reproductive health, and finding the right balance is key.

Carbohydrates: Complex carbohydrates found in whole grains, legumes, and vegetables provide a steady release of energy and help regulate blood sugar levels. Opting for whole grains instead of refined grains can improve insulin sensitivity, which is important for hormone regulation and fertility.

Proteins: Adequate protein intake is essential for reproductive health as proteins are involved in the production of reproductive hormones. High-quality sources of protein such as lean meats, poultry, fish, eggs, and plant-based proteins like beans and lentils should be included in the fertility diet.

Fats: Healthy fats, especially monounsaturated and polyunsaturated fats, are vital for hormone production and balance. Some sources of healthy fats include avocados, olive oil, nuts, and seeds. Omega-3 fatty acids, found in fatty fish like salmon, can also contribute to improved fertility.

Balancing macronutrients means incorporating a variety of foods from each group into meals and snacks. Consuming a balanced fertility diet that includes all three macronutrients can support reproductive health and increase the likelihood of conception.

3.3 Importance of Micronutrients:

In addition to macronutrients, micronutrients are essential for fertility. Micronutrients are vitamins and minerals that are required in smaller quantities but are equally important for reproductive function. Essential fertility micronutrients include:

i) Folic acid (Folate): Adequate folate intake is crucial for both men and women. It plays a vital role in DNA synthesis and cell division. Some of the best sources of folate include leafy green vegetables, legumes, citrus fruits, and fortified cereals.

ii) Iron: Iron deficiency can lead to ovulatory dysfunction and anemia, affecting fertility. Foods rich in iron include lean red meat, poultry, fish, spinach, and fortified cereals.

iii) Zinc: Zinc is involved in hormone production and regulation. It is particularly important for male fertility as it supports sperm development and motility. Good sources of zinc include oysters, lean meats, poultry, nuts, and seeds.

iv) Vitamin D: Vitamin D deficiency has been linked to fertility issues in both men and women. Natural sources of vitamin D include sunlight, fatty fish, egg yolks, and fortified dairy products.

v) Selenium: Selenium is an antioxidant that helps protect the reproductive cells from oxidative damage. It is also involved in sperm production and motility.

vi) Vitamin E: As an antioxidant, vitamin E protects cells from oxidative stress. In men, it helps improve sperm quality and motility. In women, it supports overall reproductive health.

vii) Vitamin C: Vitamin C is another powerful antioxidant that helps protect reproductive cells from damage. It also plays a role in hormone synthesis and female fertility.

viii) Vitamin D: Vitamin D is crucial for overall health and may play a role in fertility. It is involved in hormone regulation and may affect the production and maturation of eggs and sperm.

ix) B vitamins (B6, B12, and B-complex): B vitamins are involved in energy production, hormone regulation, and DNA synthesis. They support reproductive health and are particularly important for women trying to conceive.

x) Omega-3 fatty acids: Omega-3 fatty acids, specifically EPA (eicosapentaenoic acid) and DHA (docosahexaenoic acid), are essential for hormone production and function. They are also beneficial for sperm health and may support female fertility.

Including a variety of nutrient-dense foods in the fertility diet ensures an adequate intake of micronutrients. If necessary, supplements can be taken under the guidance of a healthcare professional to address any specific deficiencies.

3.4 Hydration and Fertility:

Proper hydration is often overlooked but is a vital aspect of a healthy fertility diet. Water is involved in numerous bodily functions, including the production and transport of reproductive hormones, the formation of cervical mucus, and the development of follicles.

Staying hydrated supports optimal blood flow to the reproductive organs, aiding in the delivery of nutrients and removal of waste products. It also helps maintain the right balance of hormones, ensuring the body is primed for conception.

It is recommended to consume at least eight glasses of water per day, but individual needs may vary depending on factors such as activity level and climate. Apart from water, herbal teas and natural fruit-infused water can also contribute to hydration while providing additional nutrients and antioxidants.

The fertility diet guidelines focus on the consumption of whole foods, the balance of macronutrients, the importance of micronutrients, and maintaining proper hydration. By choosing whole foods over processed foods, balancing macronutrients, ensuring adequate intake of essential vitamins and minerals, and staying hydrated, individuals can optimize their reproductive health and increase their chances of conception. Remember, it is always advisable to consult with a healthcare professional or a registered dietitian before making any significant dietary changes, especially if you have specific

health concerns or conditions that may impact
fertility.

Chapter 4

Fertility-Boosting Foods

Optimal fertility requires a holistic approach, encompassing various factors such as lifestyle, genetics, and nutrition. When it comes to nutrition, consuming a well-balanced diet rich in fertility-boosting foods can play a vital role in supporting reproductive health. In this detailed write-up, we will meticulously explore each category of fertility-boosting foods and delve into specific examples within each category.

4.1 Plant-Based Proteins:

Protein is a fundamental nutrient required for the growth and repair of cells, including reproductive cells. While animal-based protein sources are commonly associated with meeting protein requirements, plant-based proteins are equally valuable for fertility. Here's an in-depth look at plant-based protein sources:

4.1.1 Legumes:

Excellent plant-based protein sources include lentils, chickpeas, black beans, and kidney beans. They offer a wealth of essential nutrients, such as protein, fiber, iron, zinc, and folate. Folate is particularly crucial for women trying to conceive as it aids in preventing neural tube defects in the developing fetus.

4.1.2 Quinoa:

Quinoa, often referred to as a pseudocereal, is an outstanding plant-based protein option. It is not only packed with protein but also contains all nine essential amino acids, making it a complete protein source. Quinoa also boasts an array of beneficial nutrients, including magnesium, iron, and zinc, which support reproductive health.

4.1.3 Tofu and Tempeh:

Tofu and tempeh are soy-based products that serve as versatile and nutritious plant-based protein options. They are rich in protein and provide essential minerals such as iron and calcium. Soy-based products have also been linked to hormonal balance in women, making them beneficial for fertility.

4.2 Healthy Fats and Omega-3s:

Healthy fats are essential for hormone production, balance, and overall reproductive health. Particularly omega-3 fatty acids have been linked to better reproductive results. Let's look at some healthy fats that can increase fertility:

4.2.1 Avocado:

Avocados are renowned for their high content of monounsaturated fats, which promote hormone regulation and support reproductive health. Additionally, avocados are a rich source of vitamin E, potassium, and folate, all of which contribute to fertility optimization.

4.2.2 Nuts and Seeds:

Nuts and seeds are not only delicious but also provide a wealth of fertility-boosting healthy fats and omega-3 fatty acids. Almonds, walnuts, flaxseeds, and chia seeds are excellent examples. These nutrient powerhouses also deliver protein, fiber, and various vitamins and minerals.

4.2.3 Olive Oil:

Extra virgin olive oil is a highly regarded healthy fat. It contains monounsaturated fats, antioxidants, and anti-inflammatory properties, making it a favorable choice for fertility. Whether used for cooking or as a dressing for salads, olive oil can enhance the nutritional profile of your meals.

4.3 Colorful Fruits and Vegetables:

Colorful fruits and vegetables are packed with antioxidants, vitamins, minerals, and fiber, all of which contribute to reproductive health. Let's take a closer look at some fertility-boosting examples:

4.3.1 Berries:

Berries, such as blueberries, strawberries, raspberries, and blackberries, are rich in antioxidants. These antioxidants protect reproductive cells from oxidative damage, ensuring their health and viability. Berries are also high in vitamin C and fiber, further supporting reproductive health.

4.3.2 Leafy Greens:

Leafy greens, including spinach, kale, Swiss chard, and collard greens, offer an abundance of fertility-enhancing nutrients. They are excellent sources of folate, iron, calcium, and other essential vitamins and minerals. Leafy greens also provide antioxidants and fiber, promoting overall reproductive health.

4.3.3 Citrus Fruits:

The high vitamin C content in citrus fruits like oranges, grapefruits, lemons, and limes is well known. In terms of hormone production and general reproductive health, vitamin C is essential. Additionally, citrus fruits provide fiber and other beneficial compounds that support fertility.

4.3.4 Red and Orange Vegetables:

Red and orange vegetables, including carrots, sweet potatoes, bell peppers, and tomatoes, are rich in antioxidants such as beta-carotene. These vegetables are also abundant in vitamin C and other vital nutrients that contribute to reproductive health and overall well-being.

4.4 Whole Grains and Complex Carbohydrates:

Choosing whole grains over refined grains is important for fertility, as they provide a steady release of energy, fiber, and various nutrients. Complex carbohydrates help regulate blood sugar levels and support reproductive health. Let's explore some fertility-boosting whole grains:

4.4.1 Brown Rice:

Brown rice is a whole grain that offers a range of fertility-enhancing benefits. It provides fiber, B vitamins, and essential minerals such as selenium and magnesium. These nutrients contribute to reproductive health and support overall well-being.

4.4.2 Oats:

Oats are a highly nutritious whole grain option with fertility-boosting properties. They are rich in soluble fiber, which can help regulate hormone levels and support reproductive health. Oats also provide B vitamins and iron, further enhancing their fertility benefits.

4.4.3 Quinoa:

Quinoa, mentioned earlier as a plant-based protein source, is also considered a whole grain. It offers complex carbohydrates, fiber, and various micronutrients. Quinoa's nutrient density and complete protein profile make it a valuable addition to a fertility-optimizing diet.

4.5 Dairy and Alternatives:

Dairy products are often associated with calcium and vitamin D, both of which are important for bone health. However, lactose intolerance or dietary preferences may necessitate the exploration of dairy alternatives. Here's a closer look at fertility-boosting dairy and alternatives:

4.5.1 Milk and Yogurt:

Low-fat or non-fat milk and yogurt are excellent sources of calcium, vitamin D, and protein. These nutrients are essential for reproductive health and contribute to the overall nutritional profile needed for fertility optimization. Yogurt, in particular, also provides beneficial probiotics.

4.5.2 Cheese:

Cheese can be enjoyed in moderation as a source of protein and calcium. It is important to opt for lower-fat options and consume it in moderation due to its high calorie content. Incorporating cheese into a balanced diet can contribute to meeting nutritional needs for fertility support.

4.5.3 Dairy Alternatives:

Fortified plant-based milk alternatives, such as almond milk, soy milk, or oat milk, offer a viable option for those who follow a dairy-free lifestyle. These alternatives can provide calcium, vitamin D, and other essential nutrients, provided they are fortified to match the nutritional content of dairy milk.

4.6 Superfoods for Fertility:

While the term "superfood" does not have a strict definition, certain foods have gained attention for their potential fertility-boosting properties. Here are some notable examples:

4.6.1 Maca:

Maca root powder, derived from a plant native to Peru, has long been used to enhance fertility. It is believed to support hormone balance, which is vital for reproductive health. Maca is available in powder form and can be incorporated into smoothies, baked goods, or other recipes.

4.6.2 Bee Pollen:

Bee pollen is a nutrient-rich substance derived from the pollen collected by bees. It is known to be rich in vitamins, minerals, enzymes, and antioxidants. Bee pollen has been used to improve reproductive health and boost fertility, although further scientific research is needed to fully understand its potential effects.

4.6.3 Royal Jelly:

Royal jelly is another bee-derived product that has gained attention for its potential fertility benefits. It is a nutrient-rich substance produced by worker bees to feed the queen bee. Royal jelly is believed to support hormonal balance and reproductive health, although more scientific evidence is required to confirm its efficacy.

4.6.4 Pomegranate:

Pomegranates have been associated with improved fertility outcomes. They are rich in antioxidants, particularly polyphenols, which have been linked to improved sperm quality and ovarian health in women. Consuming pomegranates or incorporating them into juices, salads, or other dishes can be a flavorful way to enhance fertility.

4.6.5 Green Tea:

Green tea is renowned for its high antioxidant content, particularly catechins. These compounds have been linked to improved fertility outcomes. Green tea is also a lower-caffeine alternative to coffee, making it a favorable choice for those aiming to optimize their reproductive health.

A comprehensive approach to fertility includes a balanced diet consisting of fertility-boosting foods. Plant-based proteins, healthy fats and omega-3s, colorful fruits and vegetables, whole grains and complex carbohydrates, dairy and alternatives, and certain superfoods all contribute to a nutrient-rich diet that supports reproductive health. However, it is essential to remember that dietary choices alone cannot guarantee fertility success. Consultation with healthcare professionals or fertility specialists is advisable for personalized advice and guidance tailored to individual needs. By incorporating these fertility-boosting foods into your diet and seeking professional guidance, you can take proactive steps towards optimizing your reproductive health.

Chapter 5

Delicious Recipes for Fertility

Are you and your partner on a journey to conceive? Are you looking for a delightful and nourishing way to enhance your fertility? Look no further! This chapter is here to guide you through a culinary adventure that supports your reproductive health and boosts your chances of conception.

This extraordinary recipe collection has been thoughtfully crafted with the goal of promoting fertility and overall well-being. Drawing upon a wealth of scientific knowledge and the artistry of culinary experts, these recipes are designed to provide the essential nutrients, vitamins, and minerals needed to optimize fertility.

Within the pages of this chapter, you will discover a wide range of appetizing dishes, from breakfast to dinner, and even delectable desserts. Each recipe has been carefully curated to incorporate fertility-boosting ingredients that are known to have positive effects on reproductive health.

Whether you are following a specific fertility diet or simply seeking to make healthier choices, this cookbook offers a diverse selection of recipes that cater to various dietary preferences. From vegetarian and vegan options to gluten-free and dairy-free alternatives, you'll find something to suit your unique needs.

But this chapter goes beyond just providing mouthwatering dishes. It also includes helpful tips and insights on the science behind fertility, explaining how certain ingredients and cooking techniques can enhance reproductive function. Additionally, the book offers practical advice on meal planning, grocery shopping, and ways to integrate these fertility-boosting recipes seamlessly into your lifestyle.

So, if you're ready to embark on a delicious and nourishing journey towards enhanced fertility, "Delicious Recipes for Fertility" is your ultimate companion. Let the power of food fuel your reproductive health and bring you one step closer to the joyous gift of parenthood. Get ready to savor the flavors and embrace the possibilities!

5.1 Eleven Delicious Breakfast recipes for fertility with prep time, preparation instructions and ingredients

1. Avocado Toast with Poached Egg:
This is a healthy and delicious breakfast that can help boost fertility. It takes only 15 minutes to prepare and is packed with healthy fats, vitamins, and minerals.

Ingredients:
-2 slices of whole-wheat toast
-1 ripe avocado
-2 eggs
-Salt and pepper
-Optional: red pepper flakes and lemon juice

Prep Time: 15 minutes

Preparation Method:
1. Toast the bread slices.
2. Cut the avocado in half, remove the pit and scoop out the flesh into a bowl. Mash the avocado with a fork.
3. Bring a small pot of water to a boil and reduce the heat to a simmer. Crack the eggs into a bowl and

carefully slide them into the water. Poach for 3-4 minutes.

4. Spread the mashed avocado onto the toast slices and top with the poached eggs. Sprinkle it with salt, pepper, and optional red pepper flakes and lemon juice.

2. Overnight Oats:
This is a great breakfast to prepare ahead of time, as it takes no time to put together in the morning. It's full of fiber, healthy fats, and vitamins that can help boost fertility.

Ingredients:
-1/2 cup rolled Oats
-1/2 cup Milk
-1/4 cup Greek Yogurt
-1/2 teaspoon Honey
-1/4 teaspoon Vanilla Extract
-Optional: fresh fruits and nuts

Prep Time: 10 minutes + overnight

Preparation Method:
1. In a bowl, combine the oats, milk, yogurt, honey and vanilla extract.
2. Mix until all ingredients are well combined.

3. Cover the bowl and let it sit in the refrigerator overnight.
4. In the morning, add the desired toppings such as fresh fruits and nuts. Enjoy!

3. Pumpkin Spice Smoothie:

This smoothie is a great source of vitamins and minerals that can help boost fertility. It's creamy, delicious, and ready in minutes.

Ingredients:
-1 cup pumpkin puree
-1 banana
-1/2 cup almond milk
-1/4 teaspoon ground cinnamon
-1/4 teaspoon ground nutmeg
-1/4 teaspoon ground ginger

Prep Time: 5 minutes

Preparation Method:
1. Place all ingredients in a blender and blend until smooth.
2. Serve immediately.

4. Egg and Spinach Frittata:

This is a great breakfast option that's packed with protein, healthy fats, and vitamins. It can be enjoyed hot or cold and it takes only 25 minutes to make.

Ingredients:
-2 tablespoons olive oil
-1/2 onion, chopped
-3 cloves garlic, minced
-2 cups fresh spinach
-6 eggs
-Salt and pepper
-1/4 cup grated cheese

Prep Time: 25 minutes

Preparation Method:
1. Preheat the oven to 350°F.
2. Heat the olive oil in a large oven-safe skillet over medium heat. Add the onion and garlic and cook for 5 minutes.
3. Add the spinach and cook until wilted, about 3 minutes.
4. In a separate bowl, whisk the eggs and season with salt and pepper.
5. Pour the eggs over the spinach and onion mixture and sprinkle with cheese.
6. Bake in the preheated oven for 15 minutes.
7. Let cool for 5 minutes before serving.

5. Egg and Vegetable Breakfast Burrito:

This is a quick and delicious breakfast option that's packed with protein, healthy fats, and vitamins. It takes only 15 minutes to make and can be enjoyed hot or cold.

Ingredients:
-1 tablespoon olive oil
-1/2 cup chopped bell peppers
-1/2 cup chopped onions
-1/2 cup chopped mushrooms
-3 eggs
-Salt and pepper
-4 whole-wheat tortillas
-Optional: salsa

Prep Time: 15 minutes

Preparation Method:
1. Heat the olive oil in a large skillet over medium heat.
2. Add the bell peppers, onions, and mushrooms and cook for 5 minutes.
3. In a separate bowl, whisk the eggs and season with salt and pepper.
4. Pour the eggs into the skillet and cook until just set, about 3 minutes.
5. Divide the egg mixture among the tortillas and top with salsa, if desired.

6. Roll up the tortillas and enjoy.

6. Banana Walnut Pancakes:
These pancakes are a delicious and healthy breakfast option that's packed with protein, healthy fats, and vitamins. It takes only 20 minutes to make and can be enjoyed hot or cold.

Ingredients:
-1 cup all-purpose flour
-2 teaspoons baking powder
-1/2 teaspoon salt
-1 ripe banana
-1 cup milk
-1 egg
-2 tablespoons melted butter
-1/4 cup chopped walnuts

Prep Time: 20 minutes

Preparation Method:
1. In a large bowl, whisk together the flour, baking powder, and salt.
2. In a separate bowl, mash the banana and mix with the milk and egg.
3. Pour the wet ingredients into the dry ingredients and mix until just combined.

4. Heat a large skillet over medium heat and brush with melted butter.

5. Pour 1/4 cup of batter onto the skillet and sprinkle with walnuts.

6. Cook until bubbles form on the surface, about 2 minutes. Flip and cook for an additional 1-2 minutes.

7. Repeat with the remaining batter and enjoy.

7. Banana Peanut Butter Oat Muffins:

These muffins are a great source of protein, healthy fats, and vitamins that can help boost fertility. They take only 30 minutes to make and can be enjoyed hot or cold.

Ingredients:
-1 cup rolled oats
-1 ripe banana
-1/2 cup peanut butter
-1/4 cup honey
-1/2 teaspoon baking powder
-1/4 teaspoon baking soda
-1/4 teaspoon salt
-1 egg
-1/2 cup milk

Prep Time: 30 minutes

Preparation Method:
1. Preheat the oven to 350°F.
2. In a large bowl, combine the oats, banana, peanut butter, honey, baking powder, baking soda, and salt.
3. In a separate bowl, whisk the egg and milk.
4. Pour the wet ingredients into the dry ingredients and mix until just combined.
5. Grease a muffin tin and divide the batter among the muffin cups.
6. Bake for 15-20 minutes, until a toothpick inserted in the center comes out clean.
7. Let cool before serving.

8. Oatmeal Banana Breakfast Cookies:

These cookies are a great source of protein, healthy fats, and vitamins that can help boost fertility. They take only 15 minutes to make and can be enjoyed hot or cold.

Ingredients:
-1 cup rolled oats
-1 ripe banana
-1/4 cup peanut butter
-1 tablespoon honey
-1/2 teaspoon ground cinnamon
-1/4 teaspoon baking soda
-1 egg

Prep Time: 15 minutes

Preparation Method:
1. Preheat the oven to 350°F.
2. In a large bowl, mash the banana and mix with the peanut butter, honey, cinnamon, and baking soda.
3. In a separate bowl, whisk the egg.
4. Pour the wet ingredients into the dry ingredients and mix until just combined.
5. Grease a baking sheet and scoop 1 tablespoon of batter onto the sheet.
6. Bake for 10-12 minutes, until golden brown.
7. Let cool before serving.

9. Apple Cinnamon French Toast:

This is a delicious and healthy breakfast option that's packed with protein, healthy fats, and vitamins. It takes only 15 minutes to make and can be enjoyed hot or cold.

Ingredients:
-2 eggs
-2 tablespoons milk
-1 teaspoon ground cinnamon
-4 slices of whole-wheat bread
-1 apple, sliced
-1 tablespoon butter

-1/4 teaspoon ground nutmeg
-1 tablespoon honey

Prep Time: 15 minutes

Preparation Method:
1. In a shallow bowl, whisk together the eggs, milk, and cinnamon.
2. Dip the bread slices into the egg mixture, making sure to coat both sides.
3. Heat the butter in a large skillet over medium heat.
4. Add the bread slices to the skillet and cook until golden brown, about 2 minutes per side.
5. Top the French toast with apple slices and sprinkle with nutmeg.
6. Drizzle with honey and serve.

10. Baked Egg and Cheese Breakfast Burrito:
This is a great breakfast option that's packed with protein, healthy fats, and vitamins. It takes only 25 minutes to make and can be enjoyed hot or cold.

Ingredients:
-1 tablespoon olive oil
-1/2 cup chopped bell peppers
-1/2 cup chopped onions
-1/2 cup chopped mushrooms

-4 eggs
-Salt and pepper
-4 whole-wheat tortillas
-1/4 cup grated cheese
-Optional: salsa

Prep Time: 25 minutes

Preparation Method:
1. Preheat the oven to 350°F.
2. Heat the olive oil in a large skillet over medium heat.
3. Add the bell peppers, onions, and mushrooms and cook for 5 minutes.
4. In a separate bowl, whisk the eggs and season with salt and pepper.
5. Pour the eggs into the skillet and cook until just set, about 3 minutes.
6. Divide the egg mixture among the tortillas and top with cheese and salsa, if desired.
7. Roll up the tortillas, place in a baking dish, and bake in the preheated oven for 10 minutes.
8. Let cool for 5 minutes before serving.

11. Superfood Smoothie Bowl

This nutrient-packed smoothie bowl is an excellent choice for boosting fertility. It's loaded with antioxidants, vitamins, and minerals.

Ingredients:
- 1 frozen banana
- 1 cup mixed berries (such as blueberries, raspberries, and strawberries)
- 1 tablespoon chia seeds
- 1 tablespoon almond butter
- 1 cup spinach
- 1 cup almond milk (or any milk of your choice)
- Toppings: sliced fruits, granola, nuts, and seeds

Prep Time: 5 minutes

Preparation Method:
1. In a blender, combine the frozen banana, mixed berries, chia seeds, almond butter, spinach, and almond milk.
2. Blend until smooth and creamy.
3. Pour the smoothie into a bowl.
4. Add your favorite toppings, such as sliced fruits, granola, nuts, and seeds.
5. Enjoy

5.2 Twenty-one Delicious Launch and Dinner recipes for fertility with prep time, ingredients and preparation instructions.

1. Sweet Potato Hash with Avocado & Poached Egg

Prep time: 15 minutes

This delicious dish combines sweet potato hash with avocado, poached egg, and a sprinkle of feta cheese. Perfect for a light and nutritious lunch, the egg gives you a boost of protein to help fuel your day!

Ingredients:
- 2 sweet potatoes (peeled and diced into 1 cm cubes)
- 1 avocado (diced)
- 2 eggs
- 2 tablespoons crumbled feta cheese
- 2 tablespoons extra virgin olive oil
- Salt and pepper to taste

Method:

1. Heat the olive oil in a large skillet over medium-high heat.

2. Once hot, add the sweet potatoes and cook for 7-8 minutes, stirring regularly, until well cooked.

3. In a separate pot, bring water to a low boil and poach the eggs, about 4 minutes.

4. Once cooked, transfer the potatoes to a plate and top with diced avocado, poached eggs, feta cheese, salt, and pepper.

5. Enjoy!

2. Salmon & Green Bean Salad

Prep time: 10 minutes

This one pot wonder is perfect for a light lunch that packs a real punch. Salmon gives an added boost of fertility-promoting omega 3 fatty acids, and the green beans provide lots of key vitamins and minerals.

Ingredients:
- 2 salmon fillets

- 3 cups green beans (trimmed and cut into 1 cm pieces)
- 2 tablespoons extra virgin olive oil
- Salt and pepper to taste

Method:

1. Heat the olive oil in a large skillet over medium heat.

2. Add in the salmon fillets and cook for 4-5 minutes per side, until cooked through. Remove from the pan and set aside.

3. Add the green beans to the skillet and cook for 3-4 minutes until tender.

4. To assemble, place the cooked salmon on a plate and top with the green beans. Add a sprinkle of salt and pepper to taste.

5. Enjoy!

3. Tuna & Kale Salad

Prep time: 10 minutes

This is a quick and simple one-pot salad that will give you a powerful fertility boost. Tuna is rich in selenium and zinc, essential minerals to help regulate your hormones, while the kale provides plenty of vitamin K to promote ovarian health.

Ingredients:
- 2 cans of tuna in water (drained)
- 4 cups kale (chopped)
- 2 tablespoons extra virgin olive oil
- 2 tablespoons lemon juice
- Salt and pepper to taste

Method:

1. Heat the olive oil in a large skillet over medium heat.

2. Add in the tuna and cook for 2-3 minutes until lightly browned.

3. Add the kale to the pan and stir to combine. Cook for a further 2 minutes until wilted.

4. Turn off the heat and add the lemon juice, salt, and pepper.

5. Serve the tuna and kale mix on a plate and enjoy!

4. Grilled Chicken & Asparagus Skewers

Prep time: 15 minutes

These tasty skewered chicken and asparagus kebabs are not only easy to make, but they're also an excellent source of protein, supplying plentiful amounts of fertility promoting amino acids. Asparagus is also full of key vitamins and minerals, and is a great addition to your plate.

Ingredients:

- 2 chicken breasts (cut into cubes)
- 2 cups asparagus (trimmed and cut into 1.5 cm pieces)
- 2 tablespoons extra virgin olive oil
- Salt and pepper to taste

Method:

1. Heat the olive oil in a large skillet over medium heat.

2. Thread the chicken and asparagus onto kebab skewers, alternating between each.

3. Place the skewers on the skillet and cook for 7-8 minutes per side, until the chicken is cooked through and the asparagus is lightly charred.

4. Serve the skewers on a plate and add a sprinkle of salt and pepper to taste.

5. Enjoy!

5. Lentil & Tomato Salad

Prep time: 10 minutes

This hearty salad is a great lunchtime meal packed with essential vitamins and minerals to help promote fertility health. The lentils are a source of complete protein, while the tomatoes are an excellent source of the key antioxidant lycopene.

Ingredients:

- 1 cup lentils (cooked according to package instructions)
- 2 cups cherry tomatoes (halved)
- 2 tablespoons extra virgin olive oil
- 2 tablespoons balsamic vinegar
- Salt and pepper to taste

Method:

1. In a large bowl, combine the cooked lentils, halved cherry tomatoes, olive oil, balsamic vinegar, and salt and pepper.

2. Mix until all the ingredients are combined.

3. Serve the salad in individual dishes and enjoy!

Enjoy!

6. Lucky Fertility Soup – Prep Time: 15 minutes
This is a delicious and nutritious soup that can be enjoyed as lunch or dinner. It is made with a variety of fertility-boosting ingredients such as mushrooms, ginger, garlic, seaweed, and sesame oil. The soup is loaded with vitamins and minerals that help promote healthy reproductive function.

Ingredients:
- 1 tablespoon sesame oil
- 1 onion, diced
- 4 cloves garlic, minced
- 2 cups mushrooms, sliced
- 1 teaspoon fresh ginger, grated

- 1 teaspoon seaweed powder
- 6 cups vegetable or chicken broth
- 2 tablespoons miso paste
- 1 tablespoon tamari
- 1 teaspoon honey
- Salt and pepper to taste

Preparation:

Heat the sesame oil in a large soup pot over medium heat. Add the onion and garlic and cook until softened. Add the mushrooms and ginger and cook for another 5 minutes. Add the seaweed powder and cook for 1 minute. Add the broth, bring to a boil and then reduce the heat to simmer for 10 minutes. Add the miso paste, tamari, and honey and adjust the seasonings. Serve hot.

7. Pesto Salmon with Pasta – Prep Time: 25 minutes

This is a quick and easy dinner option with great fertility benefits. Salmon is an excellent source of omega-3 fatty acids which can help to improve reproductive health and promote healthy hormones. The pesto adds a delicious flavor without any processed ingredients.

Ingredients:
- 2 salmon fillets
- 2 tablespoons olive oil

- 1 tablespoon Dijon mustard
- 1 teaspoon lemon juice
- 2 cloves garlic, minced
- Salt and pepper to taste
- 2 cups whole wheat pasta
- 2 tablespoons pesto
- 2 tablespoons chopped parsley

Preparation:

Preheat oven to 375°F. Place the salmon fillets on a greased baking sheet. In a small bowl, whisk together the olive oil, Dijon mustard, lemon juice, garlic, salt, and pepper. Rub the mixture over the salmon fillets and bake in a preheated oven for 15 minutes. Cook the pasta according to package instructions. Drain and stir in the pesto and parsley. Serve the pesto salmon over the pasta.

8. Chickpea Curry – Prep Time: 20 minutes

This creamy chickpea curry is a great fertility-friendly dinner option. Chickpeas contain plenty of zinc, fiber, and other nutrients that can help to optimize reproductive health. This dish is loaded with flavor thanks to the combination of curry powder and fresh herbs.

Ingredients:
- 2 tablespoons olive oil
- 1 onion, diced

- 2 cloves garlic, minced
- 1 teaspoon fresh ginger, grated
- 2 teaspoons curry powder
- 1 teaspoon ground cumin
- ½ teaspoon ground turmeric
- ½ teaspoon ground coriander
- 2 cups cooked chickpeas
- 1 can (14 oz) diced tomatoes
- 2 cups vegetable broth
- 2 tablespoons fresh cilantro, chopped
- 1 tablespoon fresh parsley, chopped
- Salt and pepper to taste

Preparation:
Heat the olive oil in a large pot over medium heat. Add the onion and garlic and cook until softened. Add the ginger, curry powder, cumin, turmeric, and coriander and cook for 2 minutes. Add the chickpeas, diced tomatoes, and vegetable broth. Bring to a boil and then reduce the heat to simmer for 10 minutes. Lastly, stir in the fresh herbs and season with salt and pepper. Serve hot.

9. Brown Rice Bowl with Asparagus – Prep Time: 15 minutes

This is a delicious and nourishing bowl that can be enjoyed as either lunch or dinner. It is made with fertility-promoting ingredients such as brown rice, asparagus, and egg. All of the ingredients are closely associated with reproductive health and hormone balance.

Ingredients:
- ½ cup uncooked brown rice
- 1 pound asparagus, trimmed and chopped
- 2 tablespoons olive oil
- 1 teaspoon garlic powder
- 2 eggs
- Salt and pepper to taste
- 2 tablespoons chopped parsley

Preparation:
Cook the brown rice according to package instructions. Meanwhile, heat the olive oil in a large skillet over medium heat. Add the asparagus and season with the garlic powder, salt, and pepper. Cook for 8 minutes. Create two wells in the skillet and crack the eggs into them. Cook until desired doneness. Serve the asparagus over the cooked brown rice. Top with the eggs, parsley, and extra salt and pepper.

10. Kale and Quinoa Salad – Prep Time: 10 minutes

This easy salad is packed with fertility-promoting ingredients and makes a great lunch or dinner option. Quinoa is a nutrient dense grain that contains plenty of zinc, iron, and other minerals that help to optimize reproductive health. The kale in this salad is also an excellent source of fertility-supporting nutrients.

Ingredients:
- 2 cups cooked quinoa
- 2 cups diced kale
- 2 tablespoons olive oil
- 1 tablespoon apple cider vinegar
- ½ teaspoon garlic powder
- 2 tablespoons sunflower seeds
- 1 tablespoon hemp seeds
- 2 tablespoons fresh parsley, chopped
- Salt and pepper to taste

Preparation:
In a large bowl, combine the cooked quinoa and diced kale. In a small bowl, whisk together the olive oil, apple cider vinegar, garlic powder, salt, and pepper. Pour the dressing over the quinoa and kale and toss to coat. Top with the sunflower seeds, hemp seeds, and fresh parsley. Serve at room temperature.

11. Mexican Quinoa Bowl – Prep Time: 15 minutes

This Mexican quinoa bowl is a great way to enjoy dinner and reap the fertility-promoting benefits of this nutrient-rich grain. It is loaded with vitamins and minerals that help to promote healthy reproductive function. The black beans add even more fertility-boosting nutrients and fiber to the dish.

Ingredients:
- 1 cup uncooked quinoa
- 1 can (14 oz) black beans, drained and rinsed
- 1 teaspoon chili powder
- ¼ teaspoon cumin
- 1 teaspoon olive oil
- ½ cup sweet corn
- ½ onion, diced
- ½ bell pepper, diced
- ½ cup tomato, diced
- 1 avocado, diced
- 2 tablespoons cilantro, chopped
- 2 tablespoons lime juice
- Salt and pepper to taste

Preparation:
Cook the quinoa according to package instructions. In a large skillet, heat the olive oil over medium heat. Add the black beans, chili powder, cumin, corn, onion, bell pepper, and salt and pepper. Cook for 8 minutes or until the vegetables are tender. In a

large bowl, combine the cooked quinoa, black bean mixture, tomato, avocado, cilantro, and lime juice. Mix to combine and adjust the seasonings. Serve warm.

12. Stir Fry Vegetables – Prep Time: 15 minutes

This nutrient-packed stir fry is loaded with fertility-promoting ingredients such as garlic, ginger, carrots, and broccoli. The combination of vibrant veggies provides a healthy array of vitamins and minerals that can help to optimize reproductive health.

Ingredients:
- 1 tablespoon sesame oil
- 1 onion, diced
- 1 clove garlic, minced
- 1 teaspoon fresh ginger, grated
- 1 carrot, sliced
- 1 head broccoli, cut into florets
- 2 cups mushrooms, sliced
- 1 tablespoon tamari
- 2 tablespoons fresh parsley, chopped
- 2 tablespoons fresh cilantro, chopped
- Salt and pepper to taste

Preparation:

Heat the sesame oil in a large skillet over medium heat. Add the onion and garlic and cook until softened. Add the ginger, carrot, broccoli, and mushrooms and cook for another 5 minutes. Add the tamari and toss to combine. Lastly, stir in the fresh herbs and season with salt and pepper. Serve hot.

13. Tempeh Buddha Bowl – Prep Time: 20 minutes

This hearty Buddha bowl is loaded with fertility-promoting ingredients such as tempeh, carrots, and spinach. The tempeh provides a good source of protein and vitamins that can help to optimize reproductive health. The combination of colorful veggies adds great flavor and plenty of vitamins and minerals.

Ingredients:
- 2 cups cooked brown rice
- 1 tablespoon olive oil
- 1 package tempeh, cut into cubes
- 1 carrot, grated
- 1 cup spinach, chopped
- 1 tablespoon low sodium soy sauce
- 2 tablespoons fresh cilantro, chopped
- 2 tablespoons fresh parsley, chopped
- 1 teaspoon sesame seeds

- Salt and pepper to taste

Preparation:
Heat the olive oil in a large skillet over medium heat. Add the tempeh cubes and cook until lightly browned. Add the carrot and spinach and cook for another 5 minutes. Add the soy sauce and toss to combine. Serve the tempeh over the cooked brown rice. Top with the fresh herbs, sesame seeds, and extra salt and pepper.

14. Sweet Potato and Black Bean Tacos – Prep Time: 25 minutes

This recipe is an excellent dinner option for those looking to promote fertility. Sweet potatoes are a great source of beta-carotene which is important for reproductive health. The black beans add fiber and other nutrients that help to optimize hormones. The combination of veggies and spices gives the tacos a great flavor and loads of vitamins and minerals.

Ingredients:
- 2 tablespoons olive oil
- 1 onion, diced
- 2 cloves garlic, minced
- 2 teaspoons chili powder
- 1 teaspoon ground cumin
- 1 teaspoon smoked paprika

- 1 sweet potato, diced
- 1 can (14 oz) black beans, drained and rinsed
- 8 small tortillas
- 1 tomato, diced
- 2 avocados, diced
- 2 tablespoons fresh cilantro, chopped
- Salt and pepper to taste

Preparation:
Heat the olive oil in a large skillet over medium heat. Add the onion and garlic and cook until softened. Add the chili powder, cumin, smoked paprika, sweet potato, and black beans. Cook for 8 minutes or until the sweet potato is tender. Heat the tortillas in a dry skillet over low heat. To assemble the tacos, fill each tortilla with the sweet potato and black bean mixture, tomatoes, avocados, cilantro, and salt and pepper. Serve warm.

15. Lentil Burgers – Prep Time: 25 minutes
These nutrient-dense lentil burgers are an excellent dinner option for those looking to promote fertility. Lentils are an excellent source of protein and fiber which help to support reproductive health. The combination of spices and herbs add great flavor and loads of minerals and vitamins.

Ingredients:

- 1 cup dry green lentils
- 2 tablespoons olive oil
- 1 onion, diced
- 2 cloves garlic, minced
- 2 teaspoons fresh thyme, chopped
- 2 teaspoons fresh parsley, chopped
- 2 teaspoons chili powder
- ½ cup bread crumbs
- 2 eggs, lightly beaten
- 4 burger buns, toasted
- ½ cup shredded lettuce
- 2 tomatoes, sliced
- 2 tablespoons plain yogurt
- Salt and pepper to taste

Preparation:

Cook the lentils according to package instructions. Once cooked, drain and mash in a medium bowl. Preheat the oven to 375°F. Heat the olive oil in a large skillet over medium heat. Add the onion and garlic and cook until softened. Add the thyme, parsley, chili powder, and salt and pepper and cook for 2 minutes. Stir the onion and herb mixture into the mashed lentils along with the bread crumbs and eggs. Form the mixture into 4 equal burgers and place on a greased baking sheet. Bake in a preheated oven for 12 minutes. Serve the burgers on toasted buns with the lettuce, tomatoes, and plain yogurt.

16. Carrot and Spinach Fritters – Prep Time: 20 minutes

These savory fritters are an excellent way to boost fertility. The carrots and spinach provide a healthy array of vitamins and minerals that help to optimize reproductive health. The combination of spices gives the fritters a great flavor without any processed ingredients.

Ingredients:
- 2 tablespoons olive oil
- 3 carrots, grated
- 2 cups spinach, chopped
- ½ onion, diced
- 2 cloves garlic, minced
- 2 eggs, lightly beaten
- ½ cup whole wheat flour
- 1 teaspoon baking powder
- ½ teaspoon chili powder
- ½ teaspoon ground cumin
- 2 tablespoons fresh parsley, chopped
- Salt and pepper to taste

Preparation:
Heat the olive oil in a large skillet over medium heat. Add the carrots, spinach, onion, and garlic and cook until softened. In a medium bowl, whisk

together the eggs, flour, baking powder, chili powder, cumin, salt, and pepper. Add the egg mixture to the skillet and stir until combined. Form the mixture into 8 patties and cook for 3 minutes on each side. Serve the fritters with the fresh parsley and extra salt and pepper.

17. Baked Salmon with Broccoli – Prep Time: 20 minutes

This easy baked salmon is an excellent dinner option for those looking to promote fertility. Salmon is a great source of omega-3 fatty acids which help to improve reproductive health and optimize hormones. The combination of garlic, lemon, and dill add great flavor without any processed ingredients.

Ingredients:
- 2 tablespoons olive oil
- 2 salmon fillets
- 2 cloves garlic, minced
- 2 teaspoons fresh dill, chopped
- 2 teaspoons lemon juice
- 2 cups broccoli florets
- ½ cup vegetable broth
- Salt and pepper to taste

Preparation:

Preheat oven to 375°F. Grease a baking dish and place the salmon fillets in it. In a small bowl, mix together the olive oil, garlic, dill, and lemon juice. Pour the mixture over the salmon fillets. Arrange the broccoli florets around the salmon and pour the vegetable broth over the top. Bake in a preheated oven for 15 minutes. Serve the salmon and broccoli with a healthy side of your choice.

18. Roasted Red Pepper Soup – Prep Time: 25 minutes

This deliciously creamy roasted red pepper soup is a great option for those looking to promote fertility. Red pepper is an excellent source of beta-carotene which is important for reproductive health. It also contains loads of other vitamins and minerals that can help to optimize reproductive function.

Ingredients:
- 2 tablespoons olive oil
- 1 onion, diced
- 2 cloves garlic, minced
- ½ teaspoon ground ginger
- 4 red bell peppers, diced
- 2 cups vegetable broth
- 1 can (14 oz) diced tomatoes
- ½ cup plain yogurt
- 2 tablespoons fresh cilantro, chopped

- ½ teaspoon smoked paprika
- Salt and pepper to taste

Preparation:
Heat the olive oil in a large pot over medium heat. Add the onion and garlic and cook for 5 minutes. Add the ground ginger, red peppers, vegetable broth, and tomatoes. Bring to a boil and then reduce the heat to simmer for 10 minutes. Blend the soup until smooth. Stir in the plain yogurt, cilantro, and smoked paprika and season with salt and pepper. Serve hot.

19. Roasted Sweet Potatoes – Prep Time: 15 minutes

This simple side dish is loaded with fertility-promoting vitamins and minerals. Sweet potatoes are an excellent source of beta-carotene which helps to improve reproductive health. The combination of garlic, oregano, and olive oil add great flavor without any processed ingredients.

Ingredients:
- 2 tablespoons olive oil
- 2 sweet potatoes, peeled and cubed
- 2 cloves garlic, minced
- 1 teaspoon oregano
- Salt and pepper to taste

- 2 tablespoons fresh parsley, chopped

Preparation:
Preheat oven to 400°F. Grease a baking sheet and place the sweet potatoes on it. Drizzle the olive oil over the sweet potatoes and toss to coat. Sprinkle the garlic, oregano, salt, and pepper over the sweet potatoes. Roast in a preheated oven for 15 minutes. Serve the roasted sweet potatoes topped with freshly chopped parsley.

20. Egg Salad Sandwich

Prep Time: 10 mins

This egg salad sandwich is a delicious and nutritious way to support fertility. Packed with essential vitamins, minerals, and proteins, it is an ideal lunch meal for anyone looking to support fertility.

Ingredients:

-4 hard-boiled eggs
-3 teaspoons Dijon Mustard
-½ teaspoon garlic powder
-1 teaspoon finely chopped onion
-½ cup mayonnaise

-Chopped celery
-Kosher salt and pepper to taste
-Whole-grain bread

Preparation Method:
1. In a medium bowl, mash the boiled eggs with a fork.

2. Add the mayonnaise, Dijon mustard, garlic powder, onion, celery, salt and pepper and stir it all together.

3. Toast the bread, and spread the egg salad on both slices.

4. Serve and enjoy!

21. Pesto Salmon

Prep Time: 15 minutes

This delicious pesto salmon dish is a perfect meal to support fertility. Packed with essential omega-3 fatty acids, this meal is sure to boost fertility and provide your body with the nutrients it needs.

Ingredients:

-4 salmon fillets
-1/4 cup of pesto
-1 tablespoon olive oil
-1 teaspoon lemon juice
-Salt and pepper to taste

Preparation Method:
1. Preheat the oven to 350 degrees Fahrenheit.

2. Place the salmon fillets onto a baking sheet and rub them lightly with olive oil.

3. Spread the pesto on top of the fillets.

4. Sprinkle it with salt and pepper.

5. Drizzle with lemon juice.

6. Bake the salmon in the oven for about 12-15 minutes or until desired doneness.

7. Serve and enjoy!

5.3 Nine Delicious snacks and appetizers for fertility with prep time, ingredients, and preparation instructions.

1. Avocado Toast (prep time 10 minutes)
Quick and easy to make, this snack is not only delicious, but full of essential nutrients to support the health of your fertility. Simply mash one avocado and spread it on to a piece of whole grain toast. Sprinkle a pinch of sea salt and freshly ground black pepper for flavor.

Ingredients:
• 1 avocado
• 1 slice of whole grain toast
• Pinch of sea salt
• Freshly ground black pepper

Preparation:
• Mash the avocado well.
• Toast the piece of whole grain toast
• Spread the mashed avocado evenly over the toast.
• Sprinkle a pinch of sea salt and freshly ground black pepper over the top of the avocado spread.
• Enjoy!

2. Trail Mix (prep time 5 minutes)

Filled with energy-boosting nuts and seeds, this nutrient-dense snack is a perfect fertility booster. Combine unsalted almonds, cashews, walnuts, pistachios, and sunflower seeds with dried cranberries or raisins for a burst of flavor and essential vitamins and minerals.

Ingredients:
• 1/2 cup unsalted almonds
• 1/2 cup unsalted cashews
• 1/2 cup unsalted walnuts
• 1/2 cup unsalted pistachios
• 1/2 cup sunflower seeds
• 1/4 cup dried cranberries or raisins

Preparation:
• Place all ingredients into a bowl and mix well.
• Store in an airtight container.
• Enjoy!

3. Vegetable Quinoa Bites (prep time 15 minutes)
A savory snack, this bite-sized appetizer is a great way to add some nutrients while boosting energy. Cook quinoa according to package instructions and allow it to cool. Place cooked quinoa into a bowl and add finely chopped vegetables of choice. Stir in an egg to bind the mixture and shape with a spoon into small, bite-sized portions.

Ingredients:
• 1 cup cooked quinoa
• 1/4 cup finely chopped vegetables (ex. carrots, celery, bell pepper)
• 1 egg
• Canola or olive oil (optional)
• Salt and pepper to taste

Preparation:
• Place cooked quinoa into a bowl and add vegetables.
• Mix well.
• Add egg and stir until the mixture is well blended.
• Heat a skillet on the stove over medium-high heat.
• Add a small amount of oil, if desired, to the skillet.
• Shape a spoonful of quinoa mixture into a patty and place it into the skillet.
• Cook quinoa patties for 3 minutes on each side, or until golden brown.
• Serve warm with a side of your favorite dipping sauce. Enjoy!

4. Hummus and Whole Grain Crackers (prep time 10 minutes)

A delicious combination of plant proteins, healthy fats, complex carbohydrates, and fiber, this snack is the perfect way to add in some fertility boosting nutrients. Spread hummus over a piece of toast or onto a whole grain cracker, and enjoy!

Ingredients:
• 1 cup hummus
• 10 whole grain crackers

Preparation:
• Spread a tablespoon of hummus over each cracker.
• Serve.
• Enjoy!

5. Rice Cake with Nut Butter (prep time 5 minutes)

A simple yet delicious snack, this combination of complex carbohydrates and healthy fats is a great way to boost your fertility health. Spread your choice of nut butter on a rice cake and enjoy for a midday snack or small meal.

Ingredients:
• 1 rice cake
• 2 tablespoons nut butter (almond, peanut, cashew, etc.)

Preparation:
• Spread the nut butter evenly across the top of the rice cake.

• Enjoy!

6. Baked Sweet Potato (prep time 20 minutes)

The perfect snack for those looking for a sweet yet nutrient dense option, this baked sweet potato is full of beta-carotene, vitamin C, folate, and other essential minerals to support fertility health. Preheat oven to 375 degrees, prick a sweet potato a few times with a fork, and place directly on the oven rack. Bake for 20 minutes or until soft when pierced with a fork.

Ingredients:
• 1 sweet potato

Preparation:
• Preheat oven to 375 degrees.
• Pierce a few times with a fork.
• Place sweet potato directly on the oven rack and bake for 20 minutes or until soft.
• Enjoy!

7. Fruit Kabobs (prep time 10 minutes)
Create these fun and colorful kabobs for a snack full of essential vitamins and minerals. Simply cut up your favorite fruits into bite-sized pieces and thread them onto a skewer. Serve with a low-fat yogurt dipping sauce for an added touch of flavor.

Ingredients:
• 1 banana
• 1 apple
• 1 kiwi

Preparation:
• Cut the banana, apple and kiwi into bite-sized pieces.
• Thread onto a skewer or bamboo skewer.
• Serve with a yogurt dipping sauce.
• Enjoy!

8. Baked Apples (prep time 15 minutes)

A sweet and healthy snack, this baked apple is loaded with fiber, vitamin C, and antioxidants to support your fertility health. Preheat oven to 375 degrees, cut one apple in half, and remove core and seeds. Place in a greased baking dish, sprinkle with cinnamon and nutmeg, and bake for 15 minutes or until soft.

Ingredients:
• 1 apple
• Cinnamon
• Nutmeg

Preparation:
• Preheat oven to 375 degrees.
• Cut apple in half and remove core and seeds.

• Place in a greased baking dish.
• Sprinkle with cinnamon and nutmeg.
• Bake for 15 minutes or until soft.
• Enjoy!

9. Homemade Trail Mix Bars (prep time 10 minutes)

If you're looking for a portable and nutritious snack to help boost your fertility health, these homemade trail mix bars are the perfect option. Plus, they're easy to make! Simply combine almonds, peanut butter, pumpkin seeds, oats, honey, flaxseed, and dried cranberries into a large mixing bowl. Heat in a 350-degree oven for 10 minutes, or until slightly golden brown.

Ingredients:
• 1/2 cup almonds
• 1/4 cup creamy peanut butter
• 1/2 cup pumpkin seeds
• 1/2 cup rolled oats
• 1/4 cup honey
• 2 tablespoons ground flaxseed
• 1/4 cup dried cranberries

Preparation:
• Preheat the oven to 350 degrees.
• In a large bowl, combine all ingredients until well blended.

• Spread mixture into a greased 8x8 baking pan.
• Bake for 10 minutes or until slightly golden brown.
• Allow to cool before cutting into bars.
• Enjoy!

5.4 Seven delicious desserts for fertility with prep time, ingredients, and preparation instructions.

1. Lemon Coconut Macaroon: Prep time 10 mins

These Lemon Coconut Macaroons are a great choice for a delicious and nutritious fertility dessert. They are packed with natural ingredients such as unsweetened coconut flakes, egg whites, and lemon to give a little tartness. The best part is that this is a no bake and easy to make recipe!

Ingredients:
– 1/4 cup unsweetened coconut flakes
– 2 egg whites
– 2 tablespoons honey or agave nectar
– 2 tablespoons lemon juice
– 1 teaspoon melted coconut oil
– Pinch of lemon zest

Preparation:
1. Preheat oven to 375 degrees.
2. In a small bowl, combine the egg whites and coconut flakes.
3. In a separate bowl, stir together the honey or agave nectar with the lemon juice.

4. Slowly pour the honey and lemon mixture over the coconut and egg whites, stirring until everything is fully incorporated.
5. Line a baking sheet with parchment paper and drop tablespoonfuls of the mixture, 1 to 2 inches apart.
6. Bake for 8-12 minutes, or until the macaroons just begin to turn golden brown.
7. Cool slightly on the baking sheet before transferring to a wire rack to cool completely. Enjoy!

2. Bavarian Fondue: Prep time 10 mins

This Bavarian Fondue is a fun twist on the classic Swiss fondue that is sure to tempt your taste buds. With creamy and tangy cheeses, fresh fruits and healthier dipping options, you can enjoy a wholesome and delicious dessert that is sure to bring a smile to your face.

Ingredients:
– 1/2 cup Gruyere cheese
– 1/2 cup Swiss Emmentaler
– 2 tablespoons white wine
– 1 tablespoon brandy
– 2 tablespoons cornstarch
– 2 tablespoons lemon juice
– 1/2 teaspoon nutmeg
– Assorted fruit of choice

Preparation:

1. Grate the cheeses into a bowl and set aside.

2. In a separate bowl, combine the wine, brandy, cornstarch, lemon juice, and nutmeg until a smooth paste forms.

3. Slowly stir the paste into the grated cheese and mix until smooth and creamy.

4. Place the bowl of cheese blend in a double boiler and cook on medium heat until it starts to thicken, stirring occasionally.

5. Once the cheese has thickened, transfer it to a fondue pot and keep warm.

6. Serve with fresh fruit of choice and enjoy!

3. Quick Apple Crisp: Prep time 10 mins

This Quick Apple Crisp is a simple yet delicious dessert to enjoy without all the stress. With a few simple ingredients and minimal prep time, this easy to make fruit crisp is sure to be a hit with your family and friends.

Ingredients:
– 1/2 cup rolled oats
– 1/2 cup slivered almonds
– 2 tablespoons brown sugar
– 1 teaspoon cinnamon
– 3 tablespoons butter
– 1/2 teaspoon nutmeg

– 2 large apples, peeled and sliced

– 1/4 cup honey

Preparation:

1. Preheat oven to 350 degrees.

2. In a medium bowl, combine the oats, almonds, brown sugar, cinnamon, butter, and nutmeg together. Mix until everything is combined and crumbly.

3. Place the apples in an 8x8 inch baking dish.

4. Sprinkle the oat mixture over the apples.

5. Drizzle the honey over the top.

6. Bake in the oven for 30 minutes, or until the top is golden brown.

7. Serve with your favorite ice cream or creme fraiche. Enjoy!

4. White Chocolate Coconut Rice Pudding: Prep time 10 mins

This White Chocolate Coconut Rice Pudding is a delicious and comforting way to end your day. It's a creamy and yummy blend of white chocolate and coconut that's sure to satisfy your sweet tooth. Best of all, it only takes 10 minutes of prep time!

Ingredients:

– 1 cup long grain white rice

– 2 cups coconut milk

– 2/3 cup white chocolate chips or chunks

– 2 tablespoons honey
– 1/4 teaspoon ground nutmeg
– Pinch of salt

Preparation:
1. In a medium pot, bring the rice and coconut milk to a boil over medium heat.
2. Reduce the heat to low, cover, and simmer for 15 minutes.
3. Add the white chocolate chips or chunks, honey, nutmeg, and salt. Stir until all ingredients are well combined.
4. Remove from heat and let cool slightly.
5. Serve warm or chilled. Enjoy!

5. Chocolate Souffle: Prep time 15 mins
This Chocolate Souffle is a rich and decadent dessert that is sure to please all those chocolate lovers out there. It's light, fluffy, and full of flavor. Plus, it only takes 15 minutes of prep time!

Ingredients:
– 1/4 cup butter
– 1/3 cup all-purpose flour
– 1/4 teaspoon baking powder
– 1/8 teaspoon salt
– 3 eggs, separated
– 1/2 cup sugar
– 1/2 cup water

– 1/4 cup cocoa powder

– 1 teaspoon vanilla extract

Preparation:

1. Preheat oven to 375 degrees.

2. In a medium saucepan, melt the butter over medium heat.

3. Once the butter has melted, whisk in the flour, baking powder, and salt.

4. In a separate bowl, beat the egg whites until stiff peaks form. Gradually add in the sugar and continue to beat until glossy and combined.

5. Add the egg yolks to the butter mixture and stir vigorously until incorporated.

6. Slowly stir in the water and cocoa powder until the mixture is smooth.

7. Gently fold in the egg whites until combined.

8. Pour the batter into a greased eight-inch pie plate.

9. Bake for 35 minutes or until the souffle is puffy and golden brown.

10. Serve with your favorite topping. Enjoy!

6. No-Bake Cheesecake Bars: Prep time 20 mins

These No-Bake Cheesecake Bars are an easy and delicious way to satisfy your sweet tooth. Creamy cheesecake filling made with cream cheese, sour cream, and lemon, all topped off with a sweet butter and graham cracker crust. It only takes 20 minutes to make this delicious treat!

Ingredients:
– 1/4 cup butter, melted
– 1 1/2 cups graham cracker crumbs
– 8 ounces cream cheese, softened
– 1/3 cup sour cream
– 2 tablespoons lemon juice
– 1 teaspoon vanilla extract
– 1/4 cup powdered sugar
– 1/4 cup melted white chocolate

Preparation:
1. In a medium bowl, mix together the butter and graham cracker crumbs until combined.
2. Press the mixture into an 8x8 inch baking dish and set aside.
3. In a different bowl, beat together the cream cheese, sour cream, lemon juice, and vanilla extract until combined.
4. Pour the filling over the graham cracker crust and spread evenly.
5. Refrigerate for 2-3 hours.
6. Cut into bars and drizzle with melted white chocolate. Enjoy!

7. Coconut Berry Parfait: Prep time 10 mins
This Coconut Berry Parfait is the perfect summer dessert. It's light and refreshing with sweet coconut

cream, tart raspberries and blueberries. Plus, it only takes 10 minutes to make!

Ingredients:
– 2 cans full-fat coconut milk
– 2 tablespoons honey or agave nectar
– 1 teaspoon vanilla extract
– 1 cup fresh or frozen raspberries
– 1 cup fresh or frozen blueberries

Preparation:
1. Refrigerate the cans of coconut milk for 8-12 hours.

2. In a medium bowl, whisk together the coconut cream from the cans of coconut milk with the honey or agave nectar and vanilla extract until light and fluffy.

3. In a separate bowl, combine the raspberries and blueberries.

4. Layer the coconut cream, berries, and coconut cream in four small glasses.

5. Chill in the fridge for at least 30 minutes or until ready to serve. Enjoy!

5.5 Eight delicious smoothies for fertility with prep time, ingredients, and preparation instructions.

1. Strawberry Kiwi Smoothie

Prep Time: 2 minutes

This smoothie offers a delicious way to get important fertility-boosting ingredients into your diet!

Ingredients:
- 1 cup frozen strawberries
- ½ cup plain Greek yogurt
- 1 cup fresh kiwi, diced
- ¼ cup almond milk
- 1 tablespoon chia seeds
- 2 tablespoons honey

Preparation:

1. Place all the ingredients in a blender and blend until smooth.

2. Pour into a glass and serve.

2. Pomegranate Pineapple Smoothie

Prep Time: 5 minutes

This smoothie is packed with antioxidant-rich ingredients to help support fertility.

Ingredients:
- ½ cup pomegranate juice

- ¼ cup plain Greek yogurt
- ¾ cup diced pineapple
- ½ cup almond milk
- 1 tablespoon chia seeds
- 2 tablespoons honey

Preparation:
1. Place all the ingredients in a blender and blend until smooth.
2. Pour into a glass and serve.

3. Mango Coconut Smoothie

Prep Time: 5 minutes
This smoothie combines tropical flavors and healthy fats to nourish and boost fertility.
Ingredients:
- 1 cup frozen mango
- ½ cup unsweetened coconut yogurt
- ½ cup coconut milk
- 1 tablespoon chia seeds
- 2 tablespoons honey

Preparation:
1. Place all the ingredients in a blender and blend until smooth.
2. Pour into a glass and serve.

4. Blueberry Avocado Smoothie

Prep Time: 5 minutes

This smoothie is rich in nutrients and healthy fats to help support your fertility.

Ingredients:

- 1 ½ cups frozen blueberries
- ½ ripe avocado
- ½ cup plain Greek yogurt
- ½ cup unsweetened almond milk
- 1 tablespoon chia seeds
- 2 tablespoons honey

Preparation:

1. Place all the ingredients in a blender and blend until smooth.
2. Pour into a glass and serve.

5. Banana Oatmeal Smoothie

Prep Time: 5 minutes

This creamy smoothie combines the goodness of oats and banana and is a great way to start your day!

Ingredients:

- ½ ripe banana
- ½ cup rolled oats
- ½ cup plain Greek yogurt
- ¾ cup almond milk
- 2 tablespoons honey

Preparation:

1. Place all the ingredients in a blender and blend until smooth.

Chapter 6

Meal Planning and Preparation

6.1 Tips for Successful Meal Planning:

Meal planning is an effective strategy for maintaining a healthy and fertility-friendly diet. Here are some tips to help you succeed in your meal planning efforts:

1. Set aside dedicated time: Block out a specific time each week to plan your meals. This could be on a Sunday or any other day that works best for you. Having a consistent routine will make meal planning easier.

2. Create a weekly menu: Start by outlining your meals for the week, including breakfast, lunch, dinner, and snacks. Consider incorporating a variety of fertility-boosting ingredients such as leafy greens, whole grains, lean proteins, and fruits.

3. Consider your schedule: Take into account your daily schedule, including work, appointments, and any other commitments. Plan quick and easy meals

for busy days and more elaborate ones when you have more time to cook.

4. Use a variety of recipes: Don't be afraid to try new recipes to keep your meals interesting and diverse. Look for recipes that incorporate fertility-friendly ingredients and flavors you enjoy.

5. Prep ingredients in advance: Once you've planned your meals, take some time to prep ingredients ahead of time. Chop vegetables, marinate proteins, or cook grains in advance. This will save time during the week and make meal preparation faster and more convenient.

6. Make use of leftovers: Plan meals in a way that allows for leftovers. Cook larger portions and pack the extras for lunch the next day or freeze them for future meals. This reduces waste and saves you time and effort in preparing additional meals.

7. Keep a well-stocked pantry: Maintain a pantry stocked with staple items such as whole grains, canned beans, sauces, spices, and healthy oils. This ensures you have the necessary ingredients on hand to whip up a meal even on days when you haven't had a chance to go grocery shopping.

6.2 Batch Cooking and Freezing:

Batch cooking and freezing meals can be a game-changer for busy individuals or those looking to maximize efficiency in the kitchen. Here's how you can make the most of batch cooking and freezing for your fertility-friendly meals:

1. Plan for batch cooking: When you have some extra time, plan to cook larger portions of meals that can be easily divided into individual portions for later use. This could include stews, soups, casseroles, or grain-based dishes.

2. Invest in freezer-safe containers: Purchase freezer-safe containers or meal prep containers to store your batch-cooked meals. Make sure they are airtight to maintain the quality and prevent freezer burn.

3. Label and date your meals: Properly label each container with the name of the dish and the date it was prepared. This will help you keep track of how long the meal has been in the freezer and ensure you consume it within the recommended time frame.

4. Portion meals appropriately: Divide your batch-cooked meals into individual or family-sized portions, depending on your needs. This makes it

easier to defrost and reheat only the amount you require.

5. Take advantage of leftovers: When you have leftovers from a meal, freeze them in individual portions. This way, you'll have quick and convenient options available for future meals.

6. Plan your freezer inventory: Keep a list of the meals you have stored in the freezer along with their dates. This will help you remember what's available and prevent meals from being forgotten and going to waste.

7. Follow safe freezing and reheating practices: Ensure you cool your cooked meals before placing them in the freezer. When reheating, follow recommended guidelines for safe heating temperatures to prevent the growth of harmful bacteria.

6.3 Smart Grocery Shopping for Fertility Diet:

Smart grocery shopping is key to maintaining a fertility-friendly diet. Here are some tips to help you make the most of your grocery shopping trips:

1. Plan your meals before shopping: Take the time to plan your meals and create a shopping list based on the recipes and ingredients you need. This will help you stay organized and avoid unnecessary purchases.

2. Shop the perimeter: Focus on the outer aisles of the grocery store where fresh produce, lean proteins, and dairy products are typically located. This is where you'll find the majority of fertility-boosting ingredients.

3. Choose whole and unprocessed foods: Opt for whole grains, fresh fruits and vegetables, lean proteins, and low-fat dairy products. These nutrient-dense foods provide essential vitamins, minerals, and antioxidants that support fertility.

4. Read labels carefully: Pay attention to food labels and ingredients lists. Avoid foods that contain artificial additives, high levels of sodium, and added sugars, as they may have a negative impact on fertility.

5. Buy in-season produce: Select fruits and vegetables that are in season. They tend to be fresher, more flavorful, and often more affordable.

In-season produce is also more likely to be locally sourced and have higher nutritional value.

6. Choose organic when possible: Consider opting for organic produce, dairy, and meat products, especially those known to contain high levels of pesticides or hormones. While it may not be possible to buy everything organic, prioritize based on the Environmental Working Group's Dirty Dozen and Clean Fifteen lists.

7. Don't shop when hungry: Eat a balanced meal or snack before going grocery shopping. Shopping on an empty stomach can lead to impulse purchases of unhealthy foods.

8. Stock up on pantry staples: Maintain a well-stocked pantry with items like whole grains, canned beans, nuts, seeds, and healthy oils. These staples provide the foundation for many fertility-friendly meals and can save you from last-minute trips to the store.

9. Consider frozen and canned options: Frozen fruits and vegetables can be just as nutritious as fresh ones, as they are often picked at their peak and quickly frozen. Canned options like beans, tomatoes, and fish can be convenient additions to

your pantry, but be mindful of added sodium or sugar.

10. Stick to your list: Avoid impulse purchases by sticking to your shopping list. This will help you stay focused on purchasing the items that support your fertility goals.

By implementing these meal planning, batch cooking, freezing, and grocery shopping strategies, you can maintain a fertility-friendly diet while saving time, reducing stress, and optimizing your chances of reaching your fertility goals.

Chapter 7

Lifestyle Factors to Support Fertility

7.1 Stress Management and Relaxation Techniques:

Stress can have a significant impact on fertility by affecting hormone levels and disrupting reproductive processes. Managing stress and incorporating relaxation techniques into your daily routine can help support fertility. Here are some strategies to consider:

- Practice mindfulness and meditation: Engage in mindfulness exercises or meditation to promote relaxation and reduce stress levels. Set aside a few minutes each day to focus on your breath, observe your thoughts, and cultivate a sense of calm.

- Deep breathing exercises: Deep breathing can activate the relaxation response in your body. Take slow, deep breaths, inhaling through your nose and exhaling through your mouth. This technique can be practiced anytime, anywhere, and helps alleviate stress and anxiety.

- Engage in stress-reducing activities: Find activities that help you relax and unwind, such as yoga, tai chi, gentle stretching, or taking a soothing bath. These activities can help reduce tension and promote a sense of well-being.

- Prioritize self-care: Make self-care a priority by engaging in activities that bring you joy and help you recharge. This can include hobbies, spending time with loved ones, practicing self-compassion, or engaging in creative outlets.

- Seek support: Don't hesitate to reach out for support from friends, family, or a professional therapist. Sharing your feelings and concerns can provide emotional relief and help you gain perspective.

7.2 Exercise and Physical Activity:

Regular physical activity is beneficial for overall health and can also support fertility. Here's how exercise can positively impact fertility:

- Maintain a healthy weight: Regular exercise helps maintain a healthy weight or achieve weight loss if necessary. Being overweight or underweight can disrupt hormonal balance and interfere with ovulation and fertility.

- Improve circulation: Exercise improves blood circulation, which enhances the delivery of oxygen and nutrients to the reproductive organs. This increased blood flow can support healthy reproductive function.

- Reduce insulin resistance: Exercise helps regulate insulin levels and reduce insulin resistance, which is linked to conditions such as polycystic ovary syndrome (PCOS). By improving insulin sensitivity, exercise can help regulate menstrual cycles and increase fertility.

- Manage stress: Exercise is a natural stress reliever. Physical activity releases endorphins, which promote a sense of well-being and reduce stress levels. Regular exercise can help manage stress and its potential negative impact on fertility.

- Enhance fertility-related hormone levels: Exercise has been shown to improve hormone levels related to fertility, such as reducing excess estrogen levels and increasing progesterone production.

- Choose a balanced approach: Engage in a variety of exercises, including cardiovascular activities, strength training, and flexibility exercises. Aim for moderate intensity workouts most days of the week, but avoid excessive exercise that may negatively affect fertility.

7.3 Getting Quality Sleep:

Getting sufficient, high-quality sleep is crucial for overall health and fertility. Consider the following tips to improve your sleep hygiene:

- Establish a sleep routine: Set a consistent sleep schedule by going to bed and waking up at the same time each day, even on weekends. This helps regulate your body's internal clock.

- Create a sleep-friendly environment: Make your bedroom a calm, dark, and quiet space that promotes relaxation. Keep the temperature comfortable and consider using earplugs, an eye mask, or white noise machines if needed.

- Limit exposure to electronic devices: The blue light emitted by electronic devices can interfere with melatonin production and disrupt sleep. Avoid using screens, such as smartphones or laptops, at least one hour before bed.

- Practice a wind-down routine: Engage in relaxing activities before bed to signal your body that it's time to sleep. This can include reading, listening to calming music, taking a warm bath, or practicing relaxation techniques.

- Create a comfortable sleep environment: Invest in a supportive mattress and pillows that suit your

  preferences. Choose breathable, comfortable bedding to help regulate body temperature.

- Limit caffeine and alcohol intake: Caffeine and alcohol can interfere with sleep quality. Limit your consumption, especially in the evening, and opt for herbal teas or other decaffeinated options.

7.4 Fertility-Boosting Supplements:

While a well-balanced diet should provide most of the necessary nutrients for fertility, certain supplements may support reproductive health. Before starting any supplements, consult with a healthcare professional to ensure they align with your specific needs. Here are some commonly recommended fertility-boosting supplements:

- Folic acid: Folic acid is essential for healthy fetal development and is often recommended to women trying to conceive. It helps reduce the risk of neural tube defects in babies.

- Omega-3 fatty acids: Omega-3 fatty acids, such as those found in fish oil, have been associated with improved fertility in both men and women. They support hormonal balance and reduce inflammation in the body.

- Coenzyme Q10 (CoQ10): CoQ10 is an antioxidant that plays a vital role in energy production within cells. It may enhance egg and sperm quality and improve overall reproductive health.

- Vitamin D: Vitamin D deficiency has been linked to fertility issues in both men and women. Adequate levels of vitamin D are essential for reproductive hormone regulation.

- Iron: Iron deficiency can disrupt ovulation and fertility. For women with heavy menstrual bleeding or low iron levels, iron supplements may be recommended.

- Zinc: Zinc is important for reproductive health and hormone regulation. It plays a role in sperm production and quality in men and supports egg development and implantation in women.

Remember, supplements should not replace a healthy diet but rather complement it. It's essential to speak with a healthcare professional to determine which supplements, if any, are suitable for you based on your specific needs and health status.

Frequently Asked Questions (FAQs)

8.1 Can a fertility diet help with specific fertility issues?

A fertility diet can play a supportive role in addressing certain fertility issues. For example, conditions like polycystic ovary syndrome (PCOS) or insulin resistance may benefit from a diet that focuses on stabilizing blood sugar levels and reducing inflammation. Similarly, a diet rich in antioxidants and omega-3 fatty acids may be beneficial for individuals with sperm quality concerns. However, it's important to note that a fertility diet should be part of a comprehensive approach that includes medical guidance and treatment for specific fertility issues.

8.2 How long does it take for a fertility diet to show results?

The timeline for seeing results from a fertility diet can vary from person to person. It's important to remember that fertility is a complex process influenced by various factors. While a healthy diet can create a favorable environment for conception, it may take several months for changes in diet and lifestyle to have a noticeable impact on fertility. Consistency and patience are key. It's recommended to maintain a fertility-friendly diet for at least three to six months before expecting significant changes.

8.3 Are there any potential side effects of following a fertility diet?

In general, following a well-balanced fertility diet that focuses on whole foods is safe and does not have significant side effects. However, it's crucial to ensure you're meeting your nutritional needs and not excessively restricting calories or specific food groups. It's always a good idea to consult with a healthcare professional or a registered dietitian before making any drastic dietary changes, especially if you have underlying health conditions or specific nutritional concerns.

8.4 Can men benefit from a fertility diet too?

Absolutely! A fertility diet is not limited to women. Men's reproductive health can also be positively influenced by a healthy diet and lifestyle. For example, antioxidants, omega-3 fatty acids, and certain nutrients like zinc and selenium have been associated with improved sperm quality and fertility. Men can benefit from consuming a diet rich in fruits, vegetables, whole grains, lean proteins, and healthy fats. Additionally, avoiding excessive alcohol consumption and maintaining a healthy weight can support male fertility.

Conclusion:

In conclusion, adopting a fertility-friendly diet and lifestyle can be a proactive approach to optimize reproductive health and increase the chances of conception. By focusing on nutrient-dense foods, incorporating fertility-boosting ingredients, and managing lifestyle factors, individuals and couples can support their fertility journey.

A fertility diet emphasizes the consumption of whole foods, such as fruits, vegetables, whole grains, lean proteins, and healthy fats. These foods provide essential vitamins, minerals, antioxidants, and phytochemicals that support reproductive health and hormone balance. Additionally, maintaining a healthy weight, managing stress, engaging in regular physical activity, getting quality sleep, and considering fertility-boosting supplements can further enhance fertility.

While a fertility diet offers numerous potential benefits, it's important to remember that it is not a standalone solution. Fertility is a complex process influenced by various factors, including genetics, underlying health conditions, and individual circumstances. It's crucial to seek guidance from healthcare professionals, such as doctors, fertility specialists, or registered dietitians, who can provide personalized advice based on individual needs.

Furthermore, it's essential to maintain a balanced and realistic approach. The fertility journey can be emotionally challenging, and it's important to practice self-compassion, patience, and self-care. Remember that everyone's fertility journey is unique, and results may vary. It's important to focus on overall health and well-being rather than solely fixating on pregnancy outcomes.

Appendix: Additional Resources and References

To further explore the topic of fertility diets and lifestyle factors, here are some additional resources and references for more information:

1. "The Fertility Diet: Groundbreaking Research Reveals Natural Ways to Boost Ovulation and Improve Your Chances of Getting Pregnant" by Jorge Chavarro, Walter C. Willett, and Patrick J. Skerrett.

2. American Society for Reproductive Medicine (ASRM): Website providing resources and information on reproductive health, including diet and lifestyle factors. Available at: https://www.asrm.org/

3. The Centers for Disease Control and Prevention (CDC): Offers information on reproductive health, including preconception health and recommendations. Available at: https://www.cdc.gov/preconception/index.html

4. The American College of Obstetricians and Gynecologists (ACOG): Provides resources on women's health, including information on

preconception care. Available at: https://www.acog.org/

5. The Academy of Nutrition and Dietetics: Offers information and resources on nutrition for reproductive health. Available at: https://www.eatright.org/

It's important to consult with healthcare professionals, such as doctors and registered dietitians, for personalized advice and guidance tailored to your specific needs and circumstances.